PERSUADE WITH A CASE ACCEPTANCE STORY!

How Successful Dentists Use the POWER OF STORY to Get More Referrals and Treat More Patients

PENNY REED | HENRY J. DEVRIES | MARK LEBLANC

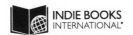

INDIE BOOKS
INTERNATIONAL®

ISBN: 978-1-952233-22-7
Library of Congress Control Number: 2020917324

Designed by Joni McPherson, mcphersongraphics.com

INDIE BOOKS INTERNATIONAL, INC®
2424 VISTA WAY, SUITE 316
OCEANSIDE, CA 92054
www.indiebooksintl.com

*This book is dedicated to
healthier patients and
wealthier dentists*

[CONTENTS]

Appendix

[PREFACE]

By Mark LeBlanc, CSP

N o matter what age you are, these words get our attention and captivate our imagination. A story well told is a story that often results in a prospect being sold. While you may shudder to think of yourself as a salesperson, the good news is selling is simply a communication process that can be learned and mastered.

If you are like most dentists, you prefer to be in a treatment room behind the chair and working with patients. You went to school for many years and paid the price for your expertise. Downtime is frowned upon: if you are not producing, revenues can slip and at times decrease dramatically.

Seldom do dental professionals study the art and science of business development. Seasoned and successful professionals from all walks of life have discovered that true, practiced growth is dependent on a person's ability to present, persuade, and communicate effectively. In fact, a dentist must understand the sales process and how it will impact the success of a practice.

In your hands you hold the definitive guide to learning why and how storytelling can be your competitive advantage in the marketplace or neighborhood. It can turn a dejected prospect into an enthusiastic patient. When a patient is enthusiastic, he or she can be the best word-of-mouth referral source. Your online reviews will be more positive, and your rate of referrals will go up.

You will discover the different types of stories that matter in your practice, along with a blue-print for developing short stories that can have an immediate impact in your case acceptance statistics. In fact, with a little work and practice, you will have a select group of stories to choose from that can be shared in your office and in your marketing efforts online.

At first glance it may seem daunting. With anything worthwhile, once you get past a little resistance, and you try and tinker with your stories, you will see how easy it can be. Have fun with it, master the art of persuading with a story, and soon you will be storytelling your way to success.

Mark LeBlanc, CSP

Author of *Never Be the Same* and *Growing Your Business!*

Coauthor of *Build Your Consulting Practice* and *Defining YOU*

[CHAPTER 1]

WHY PERSUADE WITH A CASE ACCEPTANCE STORY

Shocking statistic: Dentists are only persuading patients to move forward with treatment 61 percent of the time.

What's so disturbing about this number is that it includes cavities, a treatment that is accepted at least 95 percent of the time (2016 Dental Economics/Levin Group Practice Survey).

Here is the hard news. Many dentists might conclude the roadblock is money. Multiple surveys show the cost of treatment plays a role in less than 50 percent of cases when a patient doesn't accept treatment [Mitch Ellingson, "Improving Case Acceptance—How to Get More Revenue (and Joy) From Your Practice," July 22, 2018, www.speareducation.com].

Here is the good news: Humans are hardwired for stories. Storytelling can persuade patients to accept treatment. That means healthier patients and wealthier dentists.

Nothing is as persuasive as storytelling with a purpose. In this little book are the keys to proven techniques for telling a great case acceptance story—techniques employed by Hollywood, Madison Avenue, and Wall Street.

In addition to humorous ways to remember the eight great metastories, this book reveals how to include must-have characters into each case acceptance story, including the hero, nemesis, and mentor (spoiler: smart dentists should not make the dumb mistake of making themselves the heroes of their own case acceptance stories).

THE SCIENCE AND ART OF STORYTELLING

In August 2008, *Scientific American Mind* published an article by Jeremy Hsu titled, "The Secrets of Storytelling: Why We Love a Good Yarn." You should read the entire article, but here is a summary.

According to Hsu, storytelling, or narrative, is a human universal, and common themes appear in tales throughout history and all over the world. The greatest stories—those retold through generations and translated into other languages—do more than simply present a believable picture. These tales captivate their audiences, whose emotions can be inextricably tied to those of the characters in the stories.

By studying narrative's power to influence beliefs, researchers are discovering how we analyze information and accept new ideas. A 2007 study by marketing researcher Jennifer Edson Escalas of Vanderbilt University found that a test audience responded more positively to advertisements in narrative form, as compared with straightforward ads that encouraged viewers to think logically about arguments for a product.[1] Similarly, Melanie Green of the University of North Carolina coauthored a 2006 study showing that labeling information as "fact" increased critical analysis, whereas labeling information as "fiction" had the opposite effect.

People accept ideas more readily when their minds are in story mode as opposed to when they are in an analytical mindset. Telling the right stories, in the right way, can dramatically increase a dentist's case acceptance rates.

PLEASE CELEBRATE ME HOME

"If we want to create more engagement with patients regarding their current condition, they must be involved in the picture and the story of what is currently happening in their mouths."

Those were the words that helped Dr. Please (true story, but name changed) escape a downward spiral that could have doomed her practice.

This is the mess-to-success story of Dr. Please, who had a moderately successful practice in her mid-sized town in Texas. Several years earlier, Dr. Please had moved her home from that suburban town to a major metropolis about an hour away. Due to the commute time and missing the opportunity to take her young girls to and from school, she had reduced her patient schedule to three days per week, so that she would have more time with her family. In addition, Dr. Please's practice focus is holistic, and the big city marketplace has much greater need and opportunity for a practice with her type of focus. Her goal was to sell her current practice and relocate within minutes of her new home. In addition, due to the upcoming transition, she was highly committed to reducing her debt.

The challenge was that not only had her schedule shrunk, so had her patient base and her practice revenues. This was partly due to the reduced hours the office was open. Dr. Please was also frustrated because she had been spending 5 percent of her collections on marketing, yet wasn't increasing her practice revenues. Dr. Please knew she must get her practice back on track and generate more income in order to have her selling price after closing expenses pay off her practice debt and give her a nice start on her dream practice.

That's when Dr. Please called Penny Reed (one of the coauthors of this book). She asked Reed if they could work together remotely to get her where she needed to be and also to connect her with a right-fit company to appraise her practice and find a right-fit buyer.

"My concern is that with last year's collections, I will be upside-down in a practice sale, especially after paying broker commissions. My husband is supportive of my dream and wants me to establish a practice closer to home, yet we know we can't break the bank to do it. Is there a way to do this and what sort of coaching plans do you have? I know I need to make an investment, yet this first phase of my new vision doesn't have the cash flow to support a comprehensive coaching plan."

"Dr. Please, we can absolutely create a right-fit plan for you that supports your goal and endgame with a practice transition that generates more money to your net sale," Reed said. "We must first evaluate your numbers to see where you are, and discover the top areas that you and your team must focus on to not only help you achieve your goal, but also to get the team motivated and believing that they could still achieve their targets even though the practice has reduced its work schedule."

And that is exactly what they did.

In the initial numbers review, they discovered the number of patients being seen for their preventive hygiene appointments was lacking. This meant that there was a great opportunity, with the right strategies in place, to reengage these patients. A plan was put in place with the team to reactivate those patients, and in a matter of months, not only had the hygiene department production increased, this created more treatment plans for Dr. Please.

Yet, there was still a bit of barrier in the way of achieving greater treatment acceptance.

Reed asked Dr. Please, "How many intraoral cameras do you have?"

Dr. Please replied quietly, "One." That is when Reed connected her with an amazing resource, the website for the company MouthWatch: mouthwatch. com, which has great quality cameras at an incredible fee. "If we want to create more engagement with patients regarding their current condition, they must be involved in the picture and the story of what is currently happening in their mouths."

Dr. Please agreed and placed the order that day for two additional cameras. She also agreed to raise the standard in the office that the camera be used at each visit with every patient. This was a gamechanger.

Next, they discussed the conversations taking place in the operatory. "What questions are you and the team asking your new patients when they come in for their first visit?" Reed asked.

Dr. Please replied, "We are asking, 'What brings you in to see us today?'"

Reed called that a great question, then asked, "Do you ask them what is most important to them regarding their oral health, or what their goals are for their smile?"

Dr. Please paused and a light bulb came on. "Wow," she said. "I know we need to do that, and that is something we used to do. We simply lost our focus and got out of the habit. That is changing tomorrow."

In addition, Reed helped the team be intentional about requesting referrals and put a plan in place to choose several patients each day to specifically ask to send their friends and family. Months later, the practice revenues were up 30 percent. In addition, they made some smart revisions to her marketing budget and cut it in half. Her new patient numbers held strong and her value per new patient increased by 50 percent, due to her new treatment-presentation storytelling strategies.

At the end of the year Dr. Please shopped for a practice appraiser and a broker. Within hours of her practice being listed, she had a buyer. The transition took place three months later and as of this writing Dr. Please is devoting her time and focus to planning her new practice and spending extra time with her young daughters. She has found the perfect location for her dream practice and is making plans for her buildout and launch.

The moral of the story: patients are hardwired for stories and this can be key with treatment acceptance.

[CHAPTER 2]

THE SIMPLE SIX-STEP FORMULA

The good news is there is a simple formula for telling a case-acceptance story.

The first person to analyze the myths, legends, tales, and stories of the world and present a theory of an overarching storytelling formula that resonates across all human societies was Joseph Campbell, in a now-classic 1949 book, *The Hero with a Thousand Faces*. In the early 1970s, a young filmmaker named George Lucas, who was writing a screenplay about space cowboys fighting against an evil empire, picked up

Campbell's books and writings on the hero's journey during the course of his own research on stories and was thunderstruck to realize the film he was writing, at the time titled *The Star Wars*, followed the same motifs and structure. Years later, the two men finally met and became good friends when PBS filmed a multipart series about Campbell's life and work at a little place called Skywalker Ranch. You can't find a much higher recommendation than that.

Start with a main character. Every case acceptance story starts with a character who wants something. For your story, this is your patient—either a real one or an ideal one. Make your main characters likable so the reader or listener will root for them. To make them likable, describe some of their good qualities and make them relatable.

Introduce a nemesis character. Stories need conflict to be interesting. The nemesis doesn't have to be human; what person, institution, or condition stands in the character's way?

Bring in a mentor character. Heroes always need help on their journeys. They need to work with a wise person. This is where you come in. Be the voice of wisdom and experience in your case acceptance story.

You should build a collection of case acceptance stories that you have played a role in. You don't lead with the story; you close with the case acceptance story to improve your success rate on case acceptance.

Know what specific kind of case acceptance story you are telling. Human brains are programmed to relate to one of eight great metastories: monster, underdog, comedy, tragedy, mystery, quest, rebirth, and escape.

Have the hero (patient) succeed. In seven of the eight great metastories, the main character needs to succeed, with one exception: tragedy. The tragic story is told as a cautionary tale. (Great for teaching lessons, but not great for persuading patients.)

Give the patients the moral of the story. Take a cue from Aesop. Don't count on the listeners to get the message. The storyteller's final job is to come right out and tell them what the story means.

EXAMPLE: RICHARD'S QUEST STORY

(Here is a mess-to-success story used with permission from the American Academy of Implant Dentistry.)

Retired New York school superintendent Richard Varriale knows how to get the job done. When one of his upper molars was pulled after it had become infected years after root canal therapy, Richard could tell right away that leaving an empty space in his mouth would not be a good idea for the long term.

"It was a little harder to eat," he said, of the few months when he was missing the tooth. Anything that involved heavy chewing I had to eat on the other side. It seemed to me I was getting ache or pain on the other side of my mouth, perhaps from chewing unevenly."

Richard, then seventy-six, discussed his options with Shankar Iyer, DDS, MDS, in Elizabeth, New Jersey, an AAID-credentialed implant dentist to whom Richard was referred by his son. Richard chose to have the tooth restored with a dental implant and a single crown, rather than a bridge that would attach to his adjacent natural teeth or a partial denture that would not feel as comfortable.

"It was a simpler, cleaner, more finite solution," Richard explained. "And I didn't want to involve other teeth. Tooth-supported bridgework would have involved cutting down and latching a bridge onto my other teeth."

Dr. Iyer handled all steps involved in placing the dental implant and restoring the tooth.

The procedure exceeded Richard's expectations. "I assumed there would be some pain and to my surprise—really, it was amazing—

there was no pain other than the pinprick of the anesthetic into the gum. There hasn't been a single problem or headache involved," he said.

The new tooth has been in place since mid-2010. Richard says it's difficult to compare before and after because of the enormous difference.

"The circumstances are so changed," he said. "I now have a full, equally balanced bite; I can chew on whatever I want, on either side. It feels perfectly natural and there isn't a worry of overuse of one side of my teeth. It feels as though there's a whole set of new teeth though it's really only one. It's just perfect."

The moral of the story: Once a qualified dental implant expert has been identified, Richard encourages others to go for it. "There's little pain involved and the results are excellent."

It's not *Star Wars*, but can you see the similarities? Richard's story is short and sweet, but it still follows the formula.

Start with a main character. The main character is former superintendent Richard. We like Richard because of his undeserved misfortune—having to have an infected molar pulled.

Have a nemesis character. In this case the nemesis is trying to eat with the missing tooth.

Bring in a mentor character. This is Shankar Iyer, DDS, MDS, in Elizabeth, New Jersey, an AAID-credentialed implant dentist (ideally this is a story Iyer would tell).

Know what story you are telling. This story could be a monster story, a quest story, or an underdog story. But it is told as a quest, and the prize Richard is seeking is to be able to eat without problems again.

Have the hero succeed. Richard says, "It feels perfectly natural and there isn't a worry of overuse of one side of my teeth. It feels as though there's a whole set of new teeth though it's really only one. It's just perfect." We can see in our mind's eye Richard happily eating again, perhaps a juicy steak and some corn on the cob. In storytelling, we call an image like that *crossing a visible finish line.*

Give the listeners the moral of the story. Richard says do not let fear stand in your way. You can achieve the prize.

FIVE WAYS TO BECOME BETTER AT CASE ACCEPTANCE

To increase case acceptance, don't just use facts to tell when you can use stories to sell. Experts and thought leaders are typically great storytellers.

"Trying to influence people by using words to appeal to their intellect isn't enough," says Dr. Paul Homoly, DDS. "We need stories."

Homoly is a world-class leader in dental education. As a comprehensive, restorative dentist and acclaimed educator for over thirty years, he is known for his innovative and practical approach to dentistry. He retired from clinical practice in 1995 and now devotes his full-time focus to training, coaching, consulting, and authoring.

Here are five ways Homoly says to improve your patient-persuading stories:

Keep Stories Short. "A good way to think about stories is to picture an artist at a street fair who's perched on a stool, wearing a beret," says Homoly. "He has an easel, drawing pencils, or a handful of dry erase markers, and for twenty bucks, he'll draw your caricature. A few lines here, a few curves there, and the artist captures the *gist* of the features that make you distinct. Your mind fills in the rest of the details. Great stories are oral caricatures. A few visual and emotional words paint just enough of the picture for your mind to fill in the missing elements."

Keep Stories Character-Centered, Not Plot-Centered. "The stories you tell should reveal more about how the characters feel and less about the specific details of what happened to and around them," says Homoly. "Your stories don't need fancy plots or tons of details about the surroundings. They do need believable characters whom the listeners can picture and relate to."

Keep Stories In The Present Tense, If Appropriate. "You've probably noticed that many great stories are told in the present tense," says Homoly. "That is done on purpose, because it helps you experience the story as if it's happening right now. Switching to present tense draws the listener into the story, because your verbs are active and your language is more alive. I'm reliving it in the moment as I tell it, as opposed to narrating the past. Reliving the events in your story makes it easier for you to feel it, which makes it easy for your listeners to feel it too."

Keep Stories Visual. "When done well, the language of your story creates images in your audience's mind," says Homoly. "You'll discover that well-told stories are an auditory *and visual* experience for the listener. Listeners are actually picturing your points, which means they're fully engaged, which means they're giving you their full attention."

Keep Stories Emotional To You. "It's important to select stories that are emotional to you so you feel them while you tell them," says Homoly. "You are trying to move people to action— to make a decision, follow your advice, take their medicine. To move people into action, you need to move them emotionally.

According to Homoly's teachings, if you are not telling case acceptance stories, chances are you're not connecting with your patients at the gut level, which makes them less likely to commit to and get your recommended treatment.

[CHAPTER 3]

THREE MUST-HAVE CHARACTERS

E very case acceptance story needs a hero (think main character), a nemesis, and a mentor. If you are familiar with *The Wonderful Wizard of Oz*, the main character is Dorothy Gale of Kansas, the nemesis is the Wicked Witch of the West, and the mentor is Glinda, the Good Witch. (By the way, if we were to write the plot summary for this book and movie, it would be: "Girl arrives in strange land and kills. Makes three friends and kills again." It is the ultimate chick flick: two women fighting over a pair of shoes.)

If the first three *Star Wars* movies are more your cup of tea, then we are talking about Luke Skywalker as the main character, Darth Vader as the nemesis, and Jedi Knight Obi-Wan Kenobi and later Jedi Master Yoda as the mentors. (Our favorite mentor advice from Yoda is: "Do or do not. There is no try.")

Here is more information on the first three steps of the storytelling formula:

Start With A Hero. This is the main character. King Arthur, Sherlock Holmes, and George Bailey in Frank Capra's classic *It's A Wonderful Life* all have something in common. They are each the protagonist who propels the story. The first sentence of your story begins with the name of the main character and a clear picture of what he or she wants.

Next, Introduce The Nemesis. What prevents your main character from getting what he or she wants? Stories are boring without conflict, so the main character needs opposition from another character. Professor Moriarty ("The

Napoleon of Crime" in the Sherlock Holmes stories) is a master nemesis. So are old man Potter in *It's a Wonderful Life*, the Nazis who want the lost ark, and the Wicked Witch of the West in Oz ("I'll get you, my pretty, and your little dog, too!"). Often, the word "antagonist" is a better term. In business storytelling, common nemeses are often government regulations, the competition, or a bad economy.

Then Add The Mentor. This is where you come in. Heroes can't do it on their own. They need outside expertise or training. Sometimes they need a gentle hand to show them the way or get them back on the right road. The hero needs the voice of experience and wisdom. Clarence the Angel in *It's a Wonderful Life*, Merlin in the *King Arthur* legends, and Gandalf in *Lord of the Rings* are there to fill this critical need.

In our workshops, dentists often object to being cast as the mentor instead of the hero. "What we did was heroic—we saved that patient," they tell us.

"Ah," we tell them, "if you cast yourself as the hero, what role do you give your patient?"

The answer is, "The damsel in distress."

Nobody wants to project themselves into a story as the damsel in distress.

Patients want to see themselves as the hero who was smart enough to recognize and listen to the right mentor to help them overcome the nemesis.

Let us repeat this for emphasis: If you want to attract more patients, then your patients must be the heroes, or main characters, of all your stories (except one).

Start your story by introducing the main character—a character like your patients.

Make the main character likable.

Make people who hear the story want to root for the main character.

Next, you'll introduce the nemesis or problem. In one of coauthor Henry DeVries's stories, he labels a bad economy as "the wolf at the door." If you can use a person to represent the issue—a technique called "personification"—so much the better.

Finally, you should cast yourself as the mentor or wise wizard character of the story. With your training or advice, your hero/patient will overcome the nemesis problem. You are the voice of wisdom and experience.

A Few Famous Heroes, Villains, And Mentors To Get Your Creative Juices Flowing

HEROES/MAIN CHARACTERS

- Luke Skywalker from the original *Star Wars* trilogy

- King Arthur

- Indiana Jones from *Indiana Jones and The Raiders of the Lost Ark*

- Scarlett O'Hara from *Gone with the Wind*

- Atticus Finch from *To Kill a Mockingbird*

- John Galt from *Atlas Shrugged*

- Harry Potter from *Harry Potter and the Sorcerer's Stone*

- Eliza Doolittle from *My Fair Lady*

- Rocky Balboa from *Rocky*

- Katniss Everdeen from *The Hunger Games*

- James Bond from every *James Bond* novel and film

- Cinderella from *Cinderella*

- Lisbeth Salander from *The Girl with the Dragon Tattoo*

- Sherlock Holmes from the *Sherlock Holmes* stories by Sir Arthur Conan Doyle

- Roy Hobbs from *The Natural*

VILLAINS/NEMESES

- Darth Vader from the original *Star Wars* trilogy

- Wicked Witch of the West from *The Wonderful Wizard of Oz*

- Hannibal Lecter from *Silence of the Lambs*

- Norman Bates from *Psycho*

- Big Brother from *1984*

- Apollo Creed from *Rocky*

- Evil stepmother from *Cinderella*

- Professor Moriarty from the *Sherlock Holmes* stories by Sir Arthur Conan Doyle

- Judge Banner from *The Natural*

MENTORS

- Glinda the Good Witch from *The Wonderful Wizard of Oz*

- Jim from *Huckleberry Finn*

- Yoda from *Star Wars*

- Professor Henry Higgins from *My Fair Lady*

- Mickey from *Rocky*

- Fairy Godmother from *Cinderella*

- Dr. John Watson from the *Sherlock Holmes* stories by Sir Arthur Conan Doyle

- Friar Tuck from *Robin Hood*

- Iris from *The Natural*

- Iago from *Othello* (because not all mentors are good mentors)

THE MORE THE MERRIER IN MEMPHIS

Proper storytelling can rapidly increase case acceptance and improve the bottom line.

When coauthor Penny Reed first worked with two dental partners back in the mid-1990s in Memphis, they already had a great practice and tons of potential.

Now, twenty-four years later, they had an amazing practice and the doctors who owned the practice had their eye on retiring in the next five years. The great news is that they had two associate doctors who were wanting to buy in.

But it wasn't going to be easy: These two associates needed to generate more revenue, yet they had little physical space to do it in. Also, the prospect of having additional overhead from expanding their office hours was not an ideal solution at this time.

One of this practice's largest areas of opportunity was to increase case acceptance, especially for the younger two doctors.

They worked on communication hand-offs as well as verbal skills, and also focused on making it easier for patients to utilize third-party financing.

Within sixty days, their average operative production per evaluation (exam code), the most accurate case acceptance ratio, increased by 35 percent from $389 to $526 and it continues to rise.

The moral of the story is persuading with stories can rapidly improve case acceptance.

[CHAPTER 4]
EIGHT GREAT STORIES

First, there is a conversation. A dentist needs to listen carefully and respond appropriately. You don't lead with the story; you begin by listening to the patient first.

Sometimes you have to listen with your ears and your eyes. Here is how Tija Hunter put it in her book, *Rock Star Dental Assistant*:

> *Listen to the patient's needs and wants. Sometimes you have to read between the lines. Both verbal and nonverbal communication are huge when communicating with patients. A patient may tell you he or she is OK, but if you look at the hands, they are locked tight, fists clenched, almost what we call "white-knuckle syndrome:" their*

fingers are locked so tight, their knuckles turn white. What they say verbally and what they say with their bodies are sometimes two different things. Take time to really listen to your patient. Your patients don't know what we know. They don't know what services and treatments are available to them. Listen to what they say, but don't hesitate to talk about services they may be interested in.

After you have listened, you can ask the patient if you can tell them a story about someone who was in a similar situation. Facts and data appeal to one part of the mind, but stories are a shortcut to the emotional part of the mind where decisions are made.

WHICH OF THE EIGHT GREAT STORIES

Next, it's time to decide what story you are telling. As outlined already, there are eight great metastories that humans tell (and want to hear) repeatedly. What type of story are you telling? Almost all works of literature follow these eight basic story structures.

This chapter is based on *The Seven Basic Plots: Why We Tell Stories*, a 2004 book by British journalist Christopher Booker which took more than thirty years to research and write. The work is a Jungian-influenced analysis of stories and their psychological meaning. We compared Booker's eight categories and discovered the same rules also apply to the greatest business nonfiction books of all time.

Here are Booker's eight categories:

Monster. A terrifying, all-powerful, life-threatening monster whom the hero must confront in a fight to the death. An example of this plot is seen in *Beowulf, Jaws, Jack and the Beanstalk*, and *Dracula*. Most business books follow this plot. There is some monster problem in the workplace, and this is how you attack it.

Business book examples:

- *The One Minute Manager* by Ken Blanchard and Spencer Johnson

- *Slay the E-Mail Monster* by Mike Valentine and Lynn Coffman

- *The E-Myth Revisited* by Michael Gerber

- *Whale Hunting* by Tom Searcy and Barbara Weaver Smith

- *The Five Dysfunctions of a Team* by Patrick Lencioni

- *Growing Your Business* by Mark LeBlanc

- *Growing Your Dental Business* by Penny Reed

Underdog. Someone who has seemed to the world to be quite commonplace is shown to have been hiding a second, more exceptional self within. Think *The Ugly Duckling, Cinderella, David and Goliath, Jane Eyre, Rudy,* and *Superman*. The business books in this category discuss how people raised themselves from nothing to success—typical rags-to-riches stories.

Business book examples:

- *Moneyball* by Michael Lewis

- *The Art of the Start* by Guy Kawasaki

- *Up the Organization* by Robert Townsend

- *Grinding it Out* by Ray Kroc

Comedy. Comedy and tragedy aren't about being funny or sad; any story can be funny or sad. Comedy and tragedy are about problem-solving. If the main character tries to solve a problem with a wacky idea, that is a comedy. Think of the movies *Wedding Crashers, We're the Millers, Tootsie,* and *Some Like it Hot.* Following a general chaos of misunderstanding, the characters tie themselves and each other into a knot that seems almost unbearable; however, to universal relief, everyone and everything gets sorted out, bringing about the happy ending. Shakespeare's comedies also come to mind, such as *Comedy of Errors* and

All's Well that Ends Well, as do Jane Austen's novels, like *Emma* and *Sense and Sensibility.*

Business book examples:

- *2030: What Really Happens to America* by Albert Brooks

- *A Whack on the Side of the Head* by Roger von Oech

- *Purple Cow* by Seth Godin

- *How I Lost My Virginity* by Sir Richard Branson

- *Swim with the Sharks Without Getting Eaten Alive* by Harvey Mackay

Tragedy. This story is about solving a problem by going against the laws of nature, society, or God. Through some flaw or lack of self-understanding, a character is increasingly drawn into a fatal course of action, which inexorably leads to disaster. *King Lear, Othello, The Godfather, The Great Gatsby, Madame Bovary, The Picture of Dorian Gray, Breaking*

Bad, Scarface, and *Bonnie and Clyde*—all are flagrantly tragic.

Business book examples:

- *Too Big to Fail* by Aaron Sorkin

- *Barbarians at the Gate* by Brian Burrough and John Helyar

- *Liar's Poker* by Michael Lewis

Quest. From the moment the hero learns of the priceless goal, he sets out on a hazardous journey to reach it. Examples are seen in *The Odyssey, Star Wars, The Count of Monte Cristo, The Sting, The Italian Job,* and *Raiders of the Lost Ark.*

Business book examples:

- *The HP Way* by David Packard

- *In Search of Excellence* by Tom Peters

- *Influence* by Robert Cialdini

- *How to Win Friends and Influence People* by Dale Carnegie

- *How to Close a Deal Like Warren Buffett* by Tom Searcy and Henry DeVries

- *The Big Short* by Michael Lewis

- *Never Be the Same* by Mark LeBlanc

Escape. The hero or heroine (main character) and a few companions travel out of familiar surroundings into another world cut off from the first. While it is at first wonderful, there is a sense of increasing peril. After a dramatic escape, they return to the familiar world from where they began. *Alice in Wonderland* and *The Time Machine* are obvious examples, but *The Wonderful Wizard of Oz* and *Gone with the Wind* also embody this basic plotline.

Business book examples:

- *The Prodigal Executive* by Bruce Heller

- *The Innovator's Dilemma* by Clayton Christensen

- *How I Raised Myself from Failure to Success in Selling* by Frank Bettger

Rebirth. There is a mounting sense of threat as a dark force approaches the hero until it emerges completely, holding the hero in its deadly grip. Only after a time, when the dark force has triumphed, does the reversal take place. The hero is redeemed, usually through the life-giving power of love. Many fairytales take this shape. Think *American Hustle, Beauty and the Beast, A Christmas Carol,* and *It's a Wonderful Life.*

Business book examples:

- *Out of Crisis* by W. Edwards Deming

- *Reengineering the Corporation* by Michael Hammer and James Champy

- *Seabiscuit* by Lauren Hillenbrand (technically a sports memoir)

Mystery. In his book, Booker adds an eighth plot, a newcomer that appeared from the time of Edgar Allan Poe. From the Sherlock Holmes stories to the *CSI* TV series franchise, this basic plot involves solving a riddle and has gained immense popularity since the mid-1800s. Think of *Atlas Shrugged* by Ayn Rand and the question, "Who is John Galt?"

Business book examples:

- *Good to Great* by Jim Collins

- *Think and Grow Rich* by Napoleon Hill

- *The Secret* by Rhonda Byrne

- *Who Moved My Cheese?* by Spencer Johnson

- *The Monk and the Riddle* by Randy Komisar with Kent Lineback

- *Cracking the Personality Code* by Dana and Ellen Borowka

WHAT'S NEXT?

To improve your understanding and get your creative gears turning, the next eight chapters give you more examples of the eight great stories.

EVERY SMILE TELLS A STORY

By Michael A. Smith, DDS

One of the things I love about dentistry is the variety of people I have the ability to come in contact with in my Germantown, Tennessee dental practice. I've found that people not only have a story to tell about who they are and their life, but their smile also tells a story. That smile story may be a simple one that involves very few issues or restorations, or quite complex, involving many types of dental issues and years of treatment.

In many instances, patients have delayed treatment for a variety of issues. The issues range from the concern that dentistry is expensive, that it may be uncomfortable, or that it will take a lot of time out of their busy schedules. While we realize that dentistry is an investment, we work with all of our patients to help them choose treatment plan options that best fit their goals and their budgets.

I want to share some of the latest solutions we have implemented in my practice to solve some of the challenges that our patients have faced in their smile stories.

Same-Visit Dentistry With CEREC

As the economy has changed over the past few years, we work with many professionals who face the challenge of time away from work. The overall challenge for most patients is the thought of multiple lengthy appointments. Several years ago, I integrated the CEREC CAD/CAM system in my practice. This allows us to do many restorations, such as crowns, veneers, inlays, and onlays in one visit. What this means is that a patient can come in today with a broken tooth needing a crown, and we can prep the tooth for the crown and actually mill the porcelain crown in our office with a minimal wait. There is no second visit needed and no discomfort that wearing a temporary crown for several weeks might bring.

Sedation Dentistry

When some patients share their smile story, it is evident that they have many dental fears. Some of these may be from past experiences. Other patients share that they have never really had a bad experience, but they have always been apprehensive about dental treatment. Our office is designed for the comfort of apprehensive patients. From the layout of the office, to the decor of the surroundings and the music piped throughout the building, everything is geared toward patient comfort. A few years ago I attended a DOCS (Dental Oral Conscious Sedation) program and became certified with that system. In addition to nitrous oxide gas and traditional local anesthesia, we can offer a variety of options to make a patient's dental visit as comfortable as possible. Our goal is to add a chapter to this type of patient smile story that is a positive treatment result as well as a pleasant experience during the visit.

Tooth Replacement With Dental Implants

Most of the dental patients we see never planned on losing a permanent tooth. Yet sometimes after an injury, large area of decay, or fractured tooth, the decision was made to remove the tooth. This may have left the patient with empty spaces, or perhaps they chose a bridge or partial to fill the gaps. More and more patients are asking about dental implants to replace single teeth or to add more stability so they can avoid a removable partial or full denture.

While a partial or full denture may be the best solution for some patients, others, such as business professionals, may find that the removable prosthetic impairs the sound of their speech or makes them self-conscious.

Dental implants, in many cases, can be placed and restored in our practice. In order to provide the best diagnosis and treatment plan recommendation for our patients, we are able to do a cone beam scan in our office. This 3-D imaging software allows us to see the bone and tissue and review these images with patients to show them the reason behind the recommended treatment and if dental implants are a good solution for solving their missing teeth challenges.

Securing Dentures With Mini Implants

Many patients have thought getting dentures might be the end of their smile story; truly it is only another chapter. While dentures solve several challenges and allow many patients the ability to eat a fairly normal diet, some patients aren't pleased with the fit of their denture.

Loose dentures and partials may have a variety of causes. In some cases, the tissue continues to shrink after the denture is made and it simply needs to be relined. In other situations mini implants, like the ones we use from 3M, are a great solution to secure a denture or partial and keep it in place. This is another scenario where the cone beam scan can show us the probability of success with the mini implants and where to place them in order to give the patients the best results in securing their removable prosthetic.

Discovering Your Smile Story

Every day we see new patients who may not be fully aware of their smile story. After we visit with a new patient, we use the intraoral camera to show what is going on in his or her mouth. Most new patients comment that they have never seen their teeth and gums from that perspective. Our patients love being able to see what is going on in their mouths and know they can trust my diagnosis because they can see it for themselves.

Perhaps in reading this, you have thought about your own smile story.

It is an exciting time to be a dentist. We have so many tools available to help patients achieve the aesthetics and function they desire.

Are you happy with your smile? We would love to help you with the next chapter of your smile story.

[CHAPTER 5]
MONSTER STORIES

There is a horrifying monster that must be killed. This is a kill-or-be-killed situation. Nothing matters more than overcoming the monster. Here is an example from Penny Reed:

Case acceptance and patient engagement can be a monster problem.

Back in 2016 when Dr. Peak (true story, but details changed to protect confidentiality) hired an associate dentist, she thought it was a dream come true. Soon she discovered it was a nightmare.

While the office was busier, Dr. Peak realized she was bleeding red ink. She was fulfilled by the dentistry, but felt she was working too hard. She lacked cash flow and time to enjoy it. She was horrified that when she added an associate and another administrative team member, she was earning less than she had been before she expanded the team. At this rate it would kill the business.

That's when Dr. Peak met Penny Reed, coauthor of this book.

"All I am looking for is help replacing an administrative team member who is retiring," began Dr. Peak. Reed quizzed her regarding the real state of her practice and her goals.

"My dream goal is to collect $1.5 million per year and prepare my practice for sale, but that feels like a pipe dream," said Dr. Peak.

"You can do that, but it is not going to be easy and you are going to need to make some changes," Reed said. "Your real problem here is case acceptance and patient engagement."

Dr. Peak doubted anything could be done to improve case acceptance, but she was willing to try.

The problem was not the new hires; it was the lack of proven systems. Through the increased use of the intraoral camera, as well as improved verbal and scheduling skills, changes began to happen.

Helping the patients visualize positive results through persuasive true storytelling helped. Restorative cases, operation production, and hygiene production all began to rise.

With some hard work, her case acceptance went from a value of $566 per evaluation in 2017 to $704 per evaluation—an increase of 24 percent.

Those changes fell to the bottom line.

She gave me a call at the end of 2018. "When I just looked at my QuickBooks P&L statement, I was amazed to read the gross revenue line. We *did it—my practice reached the $1.5 million revenue goal."*

Case acceptance and patient engagement continue to rise. The practice is on track to collect $1.8 million in 2019. Even better: as of this writing Dr. Peak is entertaining multiple offers to sell her practice and remain on staff for a few years at a reduced number of working days.

The moral of the story: Your stories matter when it comes to case acceptance.

CLASSIC EXAMPLES

Monster problem stories are a staple of literature, plays, and films. Here are a few examples:

Jaws (novel by Peter Benchley, film by Steven Spielberg). It's a hot summer on Amity Island, a small community whose main business is beach tourism. When new sheriff Martin Brody (main character) discovers the remains of a shark attack victim, his first inclination is to close the beaches to swimmers. That would be bad for the beach tourism and the idea doesn't sit well with Mayor Larry Vaughn and several of the local businessmen (minor nemesis characters). Brody backs down, to his regret, as that weekend a young boy is killed by the great white shark (nemesis). The dead boy's mother puts out a bounty on the shark and Amity is soon swamped with amateur hunters and fishermen hoping to cash in on the reward. A local fisherman with much experience hunting sharks, Quint (mentor), offers to hunt down the creature for a hefty fee. Soon Quint, Brody, and Matt Hooper from the Oceanographic Institute are at sea hunting the great white shark. A shark is killed, but that ain't the real monster. As Brody succinctly surmises after their first encounter with the creature, they're going to need a bigger boat.

Beowulf (Norse tale from the Middle Ages). In a medieval land, an outpost is surrounded by an army. A flesh-eating creature called Grendel (nemesis) is killing off all those who live in the outpost. That is, until the arrival of Beowulf (main character), a mysterious mercenary who offers Hrothgar, the outpost's ruler, help to hunt Grendel. Beowulf kills Grendel, but that ain't the real monster (notice a theme here?). Beowulf must now fight the real monster: Grendel's evil mother.

HOW TO APPLY THE EIGHT GREAT STORIES

At the end of each of the eight story chapters, you will find a box showing you an example of how to apply the principles from that type of story to your case presentations. Feel free to adapt the example to fit your style. Or even better, develop a story of your own from your own patient experiences.

Ideally, you will want to have one or two stories up your sleeve for each genre of story types. This way you are ready for most story-type scenarios that a patient may find themselves in.

HOW TO APPLY THE MONSTER STORY

The easiest story to tell is the monster story. That is because it follows the problem/solution format. The hero is a patient who has a big hairy problem. The dentist is the mentor character who offers a solution. The reluctant hero accepts. The story ends with the hero vanquishing the problem (thanks to accepting the case recommendation of the dentist). And the patient lives happily ever after. Here are examples:

Periodontal Disease Is A Classic Monster Problem

The following is excerpted from *Behind The Dental Chair* by Robert Tripke, DMD:

None of us have patients that don't care how long they live. The diagnosis and treatment of periodontal disease receives a higher level of case acceptance and treatment than any service offered in dentistry...The only reason a patient will reject this form of treatment is insufficient funds, but because of companies like Care Credit, the treatment is not only made affordable for the patient, but also profitable for the practice.

The following is a news release from 2015:

Five Leading Causes Of Death From Dirty Teeth

A lack of good oral hygiene is killing the elderly and the ailment is completely preventable, according to a new book.

"There is an epidemic going on among nursing home residents," says Angie Stone, RDH, BS, author of the new book *Dying from Dirty Teeth: Why the Lack of Proper Oral Care Is Killing Nursing Home Residents and How to Prevent It*

(Indie Books International, 2015). "The elderly have increased risk factors for heart disease, stroke, diabetes, COPD, aspiration pneumonia, and thrush. The lack of adequate oral care increases these risks significantly."

According to Stone's research, the situation has been happening for years; the problem is only getting larger, yet residents and family members remain unaware of it. Even the caretakers at nursing facilities are often times unaware of the magnitude of this issue.

Stone's book summarizes numerous studies indicating that teeth and gums burdened with the bacteria that cause periodontal disease can initiate cardiovascular disease, stroke, diabetes, and dementia. These bacteria can also complicate the control of existing diabetes.

Stone is the founder of HyLife, a network of committed dental hygienists who make it their quest to provide oral care to those who need it the most. A thirty-year veteran of the dental profession, she has served patients as a dental assistant and clinical hygienist. Her original research was published in *Integrative Medicine: A Clinician's Journal.*

Stone says there are several causes of death that can be associated with poor oral health, including heart disease, stroke, diabetes, chronic obstructive pulmonary disease (COPD), and dementia.

Heart Disease: Several studies have shown that periodontal disease is associated with heart disease. Research has indicated that periodontal disease increases the risk of the development of heart disease. Scientists believe that inflammation caused by periodontal disease may be responsible for the association. The development of periodontal disease can also worsen existing heart conditions.

Stroke: Additional studies have pointed to a relationship between periodontal disease and stroke.

Diabetes: People with diabetes and periodontal disease may have more trouble controlling their blood sugar than diabetic patients with healthy gums. This appears to be a two-way street. Those with periodontal disease are more likely to develop diabetes.

Chronic Obstructive Pulmonary Disease: Research has shown those with periodontal disease have a 60 percent higher likelihood of developing COPD than those without periodontal disease.

Dementia: Oral bacteria in the mouth due to poor dental hygiene have been linked to brain tissue deterioration.

Periodontal disease occurs when bacteria are allowed to thrive in the mouth and create a biofilm in which to live and do their dirty work. Once the body realizes the bacteria are doing damage, the immune system releases substances that inflame and damage the gums, the ligaments around the teeth, and eventually the bone that support the teeth. The body does this in an attempt to get rid of the bacteria.

"Oropharyngeal bacteria are wreaking havoc," says Stone. "These bacteria can be controlled, and typically are controlled by most people through brushing and between the teeth cleaning. However, once people become dependent on others to remove these bacteria, the microbes run wild in the mouth, because they are not being kept at bay on a daily basis with tooth brushing and between the teeth cleaning."

Stone says the greatest risk of dying from dirty teeth comes when the bacteria in the mouth get aspirated into the lungs and the person contracts aspiration pneumonia. Aspiration pneumonia is a lung infection that is a result of oral bacteria, stomach contents, or both, being inhaled (aspirated) into the lungs. It is not unusual for small amounts of this material to trickle or be inhaled into the airway and into the lungs. In the general population the inhaled secretions have low bacterial count and are usually cleared out by normal defense mechanisms such as coughing.

In the 2000 report, "Oral Health in America," the United States Surgeon

General pointed out that total health cannot be attained until oral health is improved. There needs to be a movement to end this epidemic. While death certificates do not list oropharyngeal bacteria as the cause of death, they are most certainly the origin of many illnesses that lead to death.

"There are many challenges and this problem can seem unmanageable, however the circumstances can be turned around, so elders are not dying from dirty teeth," says Stone. "This needs to be done sooner than later. The population is aging, and our baby boomers are going to be the next generation of dependent adults."

[CHAPTER 6]
UNDERDOG STORIES

N o matter what story you tell, the secret ingredient is love. This is especially true in an underdog story.

This is how love relates to case acceptance, according to Alan Stern, DDS in his book *Enjoy The Ride.*

> *In June of 2019 I had the opportunity to hear Todd Williams speak....For twenty years, Williams helped develop the cultural training that developed the Four Seasons hotel chain as a leader in luxury hospitality...Williams clearly asserted that exceptional service is no longer good enough. "Lead with love," Williams said. "Put your passion first. Then present*

your credentials!" We were reminded by Williams that when times are tough, love is what matters most. When we look back on the awful time during and shortly after the 9/11 attack or other times of mass crisis, our society was reduced to nothing but love. Think about what happens to families when a loved one dies. In all but the most extremely dysfunctional cases, family members cast aside their differences and bond together. If Williams is correct that our most basic need is love, it follows that establishing a culture of love in your office will grow your practice, increase case acceptance, enhance your enjoyment of your life's work, and attract great people to your team.

EVERYONE LOVES THE UNDERDOG

Back in the days of legal dog fighting, the winning dog was called the top dog and the losing dog was called the underdog. People love to root for the underdog. Here are a few examples:

Cinderella (classic fairytale and two Disney movies). Although the story's title and main character's name change in different languages, in English-language folklore, Cinderella is the archetypal name. The word "Cinderella" (cinders + beauty) has, by analogy, come to mean one whose attributes were unrecognized, or one who unexpectedly achieves recognition or success after a period of obscurity and neglect. The still-popular story of Cinderella continues to influence popular culture internationally, lending plot elements, allusions, and tropes to a wide variety of media. Here is the Disney movie version of the plot (the Grimm brothers' version is more, well, grim): Once upon a time in a faraway kingdom, Cinderella (main character) is living happily with her mother and father until her mother dies. Cinderella's father remarries, and her new stepmother is a cold, cruel woman (nemesis) who has two mean daughters. When the father dies, Cinderella's wicked stepmother turns her into a virtual servant in her own house.

Meanwhile, across town in the castle, the land's king determines that his son, the prince, should find a suitable bride and provide him with a required number of grandchildren. So, the king invites every eligible maiden in the kingdom to a fancy-dress ball, where his son will be able to choose his bride. Cinderella has no suitable party dress for a ball, but her friends the mice and the birds lend a hand in making her one—a dress the evil stepsisters immediately tear apart on the evening of the ball. At this point, enter the fairy godmother (mentor), the pumpkin carriage, the royal ball, the stroke of midnight, the glass slipper. Cinderella marries Prince Charming, and they live happily ever after.

The Ugly Duckling (literary fairytale by Danish poet and author Hans Christian Andersen, who lived in the 1800s). The story tells of a homely little bird born in a barnyard (main character) who suffers abuse from the others around him until, much to his delight (and to the surprise of others), he matures into a beautiful swan, the most beautiful bird of all. The story is beloved around the world as a tale about personal transformation for the better. When the tale begins, a mother duck's eggs hatch. One of the little birds is perceived by the other birds and animals on the farm as a homely little creature and suffers much verbal and physical abuse from them. He wanders sadly from the barnyard and lives with wild ducks and geese until hunters slaughter the flocks. He finds a home with an old woman, but her cat and hen (nemesis characters) tease him mercilessly and again he sets off on his own. He sees a flock of migrating wild swans; he is delighted and excited, but he cannot join them, for he is too young and cannot fly. Winter arrives. A farmer (mentor) finds and carries the freezing little bird home, but the foundling is frightened by the farmer's noisy children and flees the house. He spends a miserable winter alone in the outdoors, mostly hiding in a cave on the lake that partly freezes over. When spring arrives, a flock of swans descends on the now-thawing lake. The ugly duckling, having fully grown and matured, unable to endure a life of solitude and hardship anymore, decides to throw himself at the flock of swans, deciding it is better to be killed by such beautiful birds than to live a life of ugliness and misery. He is shocked when the swans welcome and accept him, only to realize by looking at his reflection in the water that he has grown into one of them. The flock takes to the air and the ugly duckling spreads his large, beautiful wings and takes flight with the rest of his new family.

David Versus Goliath. The account of the battle between David and Goliath is told in 1 Samuel 17. The phrase "David and Goliath" has taken on the meaning of an underdog situation, a contest where a smaller, weaker opponent faces a bigger, stronger adversary. In the Bible account, King Saul and the Israelites are facing the Philistines near the Valley of Elah. Twice a day for forty days, Goliath, the champion of the Philistines, comes out between the lines and challenges the Israelites to send out a champion of their own to decide the outcome in single combat, but Saul and all the Israelites are afraid. David, bringing food for his elder brothers, hears that Goliath had defied the armies of God and of the reward from Saul to the one that defeats him, and accepts the challenge. Saul reluctantly agrees and offers his armor, which David declines, taking only his staff, sling, and five stones from a brook. David and Goliath confront each other— Goliath with his armor and javelin, David with his staff and sling. "The Philistine cursed David by his gods," but David replies: "This day Jehovah will deliver you into my hand, and I will strike you down; and I will give the dead bodies of the host of the Philistines this day to the birds of the air and to the wild beasts of the earth; that all the earth may know that there is a God in Israel, and that all this assembly may know that God saves not with sword and spear; for the battle is God's, and he will give you into our hand." David hurls a stone from his sling with all his might and hits Goliath in the center of his forehead. Goliath falls on his face to the ground, and David cuts off his head. The Philistines flee and are pursued by the

Israelites. David puts the armor of Goliath in his own tent and takes the head to Jerusalem, and King Saul sends for David to honor him.

HOW TO APPLY THE UNDERDOG STORY

Underdogs have misfortune thrust upon them. It is not their fault. Here is a sample story that you may share of a patient who for years had the challenges of an underdog and now has the smile he always wanted.

There was a patient named Robert whose situation reminds me of yours. Robert was dealt a bad hand in life. He had a genetic condition causing twelve of his permanent teeth to never develop. As a young teenager he began what would be a forty-year battle of trying to hide the fact that he had missing teeth and also to find a remedy for replacing them. Imagine being a twelve-year-old boy and wearing a flipper partial. It was a struggle for self-esteem, function, and appearance. In his twenties he was able to get permanent bridgework and it seemed his problems were over. Yet as he approached the age of fifty, after years of wear and lack of bone due to the missing teeth, the bridges failed. Robert didn't want a denture; even the prospect of a denture was dismal due to his lack of bone. One great thing that Robert had on his side was the advances in dental treatment over the last four decades. Robert was able to have bone grafting, six dental implants, and crowns on those implants. The results were life-changing. He can now eat, talk, and smile just like he would have if he had all of his permanent teeth. Robert says his only regret was that he waited so long to have the work done.

[CHAPTER 7]
COMEDY STORIES

I f you try to solve the problem with a wacky idea, that is a comedy. A true comedy usually ends in romance or marriage. While you probably will not be telling many wacky idea case-acceptance stories, you should know what comedy stories are well known. Here are some examples:

Tootsie (film by Sydney Pollack). Michael Dorsey (main character) is renowned in the entertainment field for being a good but difficult and temperamental actor. He is informed by his agent, George Fields (mentor), that no one will hire him because of his bad reputation. In his personal life, Michael is a bit of a cad who treats women poorly, especially his long-term friend and fellow actor Sandy

Lester, a doormat of a woman who already has self-esteem issues. Both to prove George wrong and to raise money to finance a play written by his roommate, Jeff Slater, so that he and Sandy can star in it, Michael goes incognito as female Dorothy Michaels and auditions for a role in the soap opera *Southwest General* (wacky idea). The role is Emily Kimberley, the tough, no-nonsense administrator of the hospital. As Dorothy, Michael injects into his audition his own sensibilities, which lands him the short-term role. As Michael progresses in the role, only George and Jeff know Dorothy's identity.

As Dorothy, Michael continues to play the role as he himself would, often ad-libbing. He detests his director, Ron Carlisle (nemesis) for the way he treats "her" and women in general (much the way Michael treated women himself), including Ron's girlfriend, lead *Southwest General* actress, Julie Nichols. Dorothy treats Julie with care and respect and begins to fall in love with her. However, two men fall for Dorothy, namely *Southwest General*'s long-time Lothario lead actor, John

Van Horn, and Julie's father, Les. Michael must find a way to let Julie know his feelings as a man without ruining their friendship. Worse problems arise for Michael when Dorothy's no-exit clause contract on *Southwest General* is extended, meaning Michael may have to pretend to be Dorothy for much longer than originally intended.

Some Like It Hot (film by Billy Wilder). It's the winter of 1929 in Chicago. Friends and roommates Jerry and Joe (main characters) are band musicians—a string bassist and tenor saxophonist, respectively. They are also deeply in debt. Smooth-talking womanizer Joe is a glass-half-full type who figures they can earn quick money to pay off their debts by gambling with the little money they earn. More conservative Jerry is a glass-half-empty type of guy. They are in the wrong place at the wrong time when they witness a gangland slaying by bootlegger Spats Colombo (nemesis) and his men. Jerry and Joe manage to make it away from the scene within an inch of their lives.

Needing to lay low and get out of town, away from Spats, they sense an opportunity when they learn of a local jazz band needing a bassist and a saxophonist for a three-week gig at a luxurious tropical seaside resort in Miami, all expenses paid. The problem? This is an all-girl band—but nothing that "Geraldine" and "Josephine" can't overcome by dressing in disguise as women (wacky idea), the former of whom instead chooses Daphne as "her" stage name. Sweet Sue, the band leader, has two basic rules for the band members while on tour: no liquor and no men. Beyond needing to evade Spats and his henchmen and maintain the front of being women (especially in the most private of situations with the other female band members), Jerry and Joe have two additional problems.

First, the more brazen Joe falls for one of the other band members, ukulele player and vocalist Sugar Kane Kowalczyk (although Jerry, too, is attracted to her). Joe does whatever he can to find time to get out of drag to woo Sugar while in Miami, using all the knowledge

Josephine gleans directly from Sugar about what floats her boat in potential-husband material. And second, Jerry, as Daphne, catches the eye of wealthy love-struck Osgood Fielding III, who doggedly pursues "her" and won't take no for an answer. The last line of the movie is one of the greatest in the history of cinema. As Shakespeare would say, all's well that ends well, with this comedy of errors.

A Funny Thing Happened on the Way to the Forum (Stephen Sondheim Broadway play and film adaptation, inspired by the farces of the ancient Roman playwright Plautus [251–183 BC], specifically Pseudolus, Miles Gloriosus, and Mostellaria). As the song says, "Tragedy tomorrow; comedy tonight." This screen adaptation of the stage musical of the same name finds the Roman slave Pseudolus (main character) scheming his way to freedom by playing matchmaker (wacky idea) for his master's son, Hero, who is smitten with the blonde and beautiful Philia. But things don't go according to plan. The hijinks and complications that ensue involve blackmail, funny disguises, and long-lost children. Pseudolus desperately tries to keep his end of the bargain while a Roman army officer (nemesis) could be the death of him.

HOW TO APPLY THE COMEDY STORY

The key to a comedy story is talking about solving a problem with a wacky idea. Dentistry can be so serious that sometimes you might want to lighten the mood.

When Marvin came in for his new patient visit, I remember how beautiful and white his teeth were. He hadn't been to the dentist in years and finally had dental insurance, so he thought he would come in for a check-up. Sadly, what Marvin didn't know is that while his teeth looked beautiful, and he wasn't in any pain, he was in the late stages of gum (periodontal) disease. The disease was so advanced that most of his teeth could not be saved. When I told Marvin he should have full dentures, he thought that was a wacky idea. Marvin made the choice to have full dentures. The day of the appointment came and he was nervous. The procedure went well, and on that day, we delivered a beautiful set of dentures. While Marvin was happy with the appearance of his new dentures, he looked at our assistant with a touch of sadness in his eyes. "Thank you, but I admit this has been a comedy of errors for me," said Marvin. "I wish I had known to take better care of my gums and that my gum disease had been caught early on." Nobody wants to put their teeth in a glass at night, but sometimes a wacky idea like full dentures is the only solution for an all's-well-that-ends-well outcome.

[CHAPTER 8]
TRAGEDY STORIES

I f a person tries to solve a problem by going against the laws of society, nature, or God, then that is tragedy. The decision to take a shortcut is the tragic decision.

As noted earlier, the tragedy doesn't readily lend itself to case acceptance stories. That's because it's a harsh cautionary tale with no room for hope, lessons learned, or redemption until it's far too late for any of the characters, who tend to end up dead in pools of blood at the end due to their poor decisions, or through no fault of their own.

We do not recommend tragedy stories as persuasive case acceptance; a case acceptance story is a better bet. But, to fully illustrate the tragedy story, here are some examples.

Othello (play by William Shakespeare). A 1500s Venetian general, Othello (main character) allows his marriage to be destroyed when a vengeful lieutenant convinces him that his new wife has been unfaithful. Iago (nemesis/mentor), a Venetian army officer and ensign to the Moorish general, Othello, bitterly resents the appointment of Cassio as Othello's chief lieutenant. Roderigo and Iago maliciously bait Brabantio, an old senator, with the news that his daughter, Desdemona, is betrothed to Othello. Before the Council Chamber, Brabantio accused Othello of abducting his daughter to elope with her. The Moor denies this, and Desdemona affirms loyalty to her new husband. Othello is ordered to defend Cyprus, of which he is governor against the Turks. Iago (here is the problem—Othello lets his nemesis also be his mentor) assures Roderigo, who is also secretly in love with Desdemona, that she will not love Othello for long. Iago brings

Desdemona to Cyprus to celebrate Othello's victory against the Turks and incites Cassio and Montano into a drunken brawl. Montano is seriously hurt and Iago beckons Othello, blaming Cassio, who is dismissed from duties. Iago then advises Cassio to seek Desdemona's assistance in regaining Othello's favor. Iago arranges for Othello to find his wife in earnest conversation with Cassio, and subtly arouses the Moor's jealousy by creating a slanderous piece of evidence, placing Desdemona's handkerchief (an intimate item) in Cassio's possession. Othello's fatal flaw is believing Iago's lie that his lieutenant, Cassio, has been cuckolding him—a lie that leads to a tragic end. Othello ultimately kills Desdemona in a jealous rage and commits suicide. Cassio also gets a decent stab in the leg for his pains, and when Iago's wife realizes he's behind the whole thing, she exposes him and he kills her as well. Other bodies pile up along the way. Iago himself survives the carnage and vows never to explain why he decided to set in motion all these horrible acts in the first place.

King Lear (play by William Shakespeare). King Lear (main character), old and tired, divides his kingdom among his daughters, giving great importance to their elaborate declarations of love for him. When Cordelia, youngest and most honest, refuses to idly flatter the old man in return for favor, he banishes her and turns to his remaining daughters for support. But older daughters Goneril and Regan (nemesis characters) have no love for him and instead plot to take all his power from him. In a parallel, Lear's loyal courtier Gloucester favors his illegitimate son, Edmund, after being told lies about his faithful son, Edgar. Madness and tragedy befall both ill-fated but prideful fathers. They even hang King Lear's court jester (mentor), a fool who spoke the truth to the king.

The Godfather (novel by Mario Puzo and film by Francis Ford Coppola). In the novel and film *The Godfather*, "Don" Vito Corleone (main character) is the head of the Corleone mafia family in New York. The story opens at his daughter's wedding. Michael, Vito's youngest son and a decorated World War II Marine veteran, is also present at the wedding. Michael seems to be uninterested in being a part of the family business. Vito is a powerful man and is kind to all those who show him respect but is ruthless against those who do not. When a powerful and treacherous rival (nemesis) wants to sell drugs and needs the Don's influence for the same, Vito refuses to do it. What follows is a clash between Vito's fading old values and the new ways, which may cause Michael to do the thing he was most reluctant to do: wage a mob war against all the other mafia families, which could tear the Corleone family apart. This is how Michael Corleone becomes the tragic hero (new main character) of *The Godfather* trilogy. He makes the tragic decision to join the family business. And although he says it is business and not personal, trust me, it is personal. Unsurprisingly (it's a tragedy), the body count is high, and in the end, Michael dies a broken man, unremembered and alone.

HOW TO APPLY THE TRAGEDY STORY

A tragedy story is a cautionary tale. The key to this story for case acceptance is talking about how a great tragedy was avoided.

Avoiding the dentist can have tragic consequences. The hero of this story is Fred's mom. Fred was four years old when his mom noticed a small bulge in his cheek. Putting off seeing healthcare providers is not unusual. But Fred's mom decided to take him to the pediatrician who then referred him to his dentist. Fred's mom decided to go the extra step and take Fred to see the dentist. Dental visits for children are farm ore than simple evaluations and cleanings. Upon evaluation and x-ray, Fred was scheduled with an oral surgeon to remove what appeared to be a cyst under his tooth. That cyst turned out to be more serious than anyone anticipated. Within twenty-four hours, Fred was admitted to St. Jude Children's Research Hospital in Memphis, Tennessee where he began a year-long battle with leukemia. This story has a happy ending. Due to early detection and treatment, Fred is doing well today and has just graduated from college. He is now interviewing with St. Jude in the marketing department to help save the lives of other children.

[CHAPTER 9]
MYSTERY STORIES

Whodunnit? Either the audience is in the dark along with the hero, or the audience knows the answer and wonders how and when the main character will figure it all out.

Here are examples:

The Hound of the Baskervilles (novel by Sir Arthur Conan Doyle, plus many film versions). Sherlock Holmes (main character) is a consulting detective in Victorian London. When Sir Charles Baskerville dies unexpectedly, his nephew and heir, Sir Henry, returns from South Africa. Dr. Mortimer, the local doctor, is concerned about Sir Henry's safety, as he is convinced that Sir Charles was literally frightened to death. He consults detective Sherlock Holmes and recounts the tale of one Sir Hugo Baskerville who, several generations previously, had been killed by a huge hound and which now is believed by some to be a curse on the family. Holmes agrees to take on the case and it almost immediately becomes apparent that Sir Henry's life is in danger. Holmes doesn't believe in the legend of the Baskervilles or the supposed curse placed upon them and sets out to find a more practical solution. (Interesting story fact: Sherlock Holmes holds the Guinness World Record for having been portrayed more times on film and TV than any other character.) Spoiler alert: Holmes cracks the case.

Murder on the Orient Express (novel by Agatha Christie, film directed by Sidney Lumet). Unexpectedly returning to England from Istanbul in 1935, famed Belgian detective Hercule Poirot (main character) finds himself traveling on the luxury train the Orient Express. One of the passengers, Mr. Ratchett, informs Poirot that he has been receiving anonymous threats and asks Poirot to act as his bodyguard. Poirot declines, but when Ratchett is found stabbed to death the next morning, it is apparent that the threats he had received were real. Poirot soon deduces that Ratchett was, in fact, the infamous Cassetti, believed to have been the man behind the kidnapping and murder of three-year-old Daisy Armstrong some five years previously. As he begins to question the dozen or so passengers on the train, he realizes several of them have a connection to the Armstrong family and he begins to form a solution to a complex crime. And the murderer is...

HOW TO APPLY THE MYSTERY STORY

A mystery story is about a riddle, a puzzle, or unlocking the code. Drop words like that and secret, clue, and detective work into the story to appeal to the listener.

It was a mystery to Alice, a nice woman who just turned fifty, as to what was wrong. She told us at her cleaning appointment that while mother nature may be in control of a lot of her aging process, she was determined not to give up on staying young without a fight. She wanted our help to crack the code on what would be best for her. Alice mentioned she had never been happy with her smile. She had the undeserved misfortune of her upper front teeth being too small, and they had a funny shape. She was ready for a makeover but didn't have a clue how to proceed. After an evaluation, we told her she would need twelve units (both crowns and veneers) on the upper and if she wanted the front lowers to match, she would be looking at another eight units (both crowns and veneers). She decided she wanted to do the upper and lower and was puzzled as to how to pay for it. She had put several thousand dollars away and knew her treatment would be quite a bit more. Alice was excited to hear about an extended payment plan we offer through CareCredit. She would be able to have the smile of her dreams now and pay it off in twenty-four months. Alice scheduled right away and within a few weeks her treatment was complete. She was thrilled with the results and said her only regret was not getting the work done sooner. "If I had known that I could utilize a payment plan, I would have had this work done years ago," said Alice. "I love my new smile and as a matter of fact, I can't stop smiling."

[CHAPTER 10]
QUEST STORIES

Quest stories are about a journey to find a great prize, or to use Joseph Campbell's word, a boon. Perhaps the prize is to rescue someone, recover something, save the world, or obtain some treasure. Maybe the real treasure is the knowledge you learn along the way. Many memoirs are quest stories. Here are some classic story examples:

Indiana Jones and The Raiders of the Lost Ark (a film by George Lucas and Stephen Spielberg). The year is 1936. Archeology professor Indiana Jones (main character) narrowly escapes death in a South American temple after obtaining a gold idol—death by poison dart, fall, and finally a giant boulder that chases him out the front of a cave. An old enemy, René Belloq, steals the idol and then orders a group of natives to chase "Indy" down and kill him. Indy, however, escapes back to the United States, where Army intelligence officers are waiting for him at his university. They tell him about a flurry of Nazi archaeological activity near Cairo, which Indy determines may be related to the possible resting place of the Ark of the Covenant—the chest that carried the original Ten Commandments. The ark is believed to carry an incredibly powerful source of energy that must not fall into Nazi hands.

Indiana is immediately sent overseas, stopping in Nepal to pick up a relic his old professor had that may hold the key to the ark's location (and also his former girlfriend Marion, his old professor's daughter), then meeting up in Cairo with his friend Sallah. But danger lurks everywhere in the form of Nazi thugs and poisonous snakes in the ark's resting place. After Belloq, hired by the Nazis, beats Indy to the treasure again, this time the ark, Indy and Marion are determined to get it back, and they overpower the pilot of a German plane.

But Indy finds himself confronted with a giant German thug, and after a frightening hand-to-hand fight, Indy and Marion blow up the plane. Now the Nazis must drive the ark to Cairo, but Indy regains control of the ark after running the convoy off the road, one vehicle at a time. Once again, the Nazis recapture the ark—and Marion—and head for a Nazi-controlled island. There, Belloq will open the ark to demonstrate the horrific power it can *unleash upon the world.*

The Grapes of Wrath (novel by John Steinbeck; film by John Ford, Darryl F. Zanuck, and Nunnally Johnson). After serving four years in prison for killing a man, hotheaded Tom Joad (main character) heads back to the family farm in Oklahoma. Tom is reunited with his family at his uncle's farm only to discover the family must leave that farm the next day. The extended family packs their belongings onto an old truck and drives to California to look for work. They arrive at an itinerant camp populated with hungry children. A man and sheriff come to the camp promising work but won't say how much they will be paid. The family leaves the camp and arrives at a farm that needs workers. Tom is wary. The farm is surrounding by a barbed-wire fence with plenty of armed guards. The family settles into a shack and picks peaches for five cents a box, earning barely enough to feed the family. Tom kills a thug attacking farm union organizers and must go on the lam. The family loads up the truck again, hiding Tom under a mattress. They head north and find a camp run by the United States Department of Agriculture. Life is better. The sheriff arrives at the camp looking for Tom. Tom vows to his mother that he will fight injustice wherever he finds it and heads off into the night. The family moves on, hopeful of a better life down the road.

HOW TO APPLY THE QUEST STORY

A quest story is about a journey in search of a prize of great value. There is a call to the quest for the patient, and you are the guide on their journey.

Brent came to our office in his early forties. He was on a quest for a beautiful smile. We were happy to answer the call to his quest.

"I am really embarrassed of my smile," confessed Brent. "Maybe I need veneers? What can I do to get a great smile?"

We thought the journey was not going to be easy. Brent's teeth were far from straight and had a bit of a gray cast to them. But upon examination, we found his teeth were in great shape.

"Good news Brent: we are recommending orthodontics which would be followed up

by tooth whitening to give you a smile you can be proud of," I told him.

Brent was skeptical at first. He also was not excited about having braces as an adult. Based on our discussion, he decided to move forward on the journey with the orthodontic treatment.

The quest was not an overnight fix. However, within twelve months, Brent had been through his complete ortho-dontic treatment, as well as having his teeth whitened.

He told us: "Thank you. I couldn't be happier with the outcome. Now I have a smile that makes me proud."

[CHAPTER 11]
REBIRTH STORIES

What was dead has come back to life. Like a phoenix rising from the ashes, a person or institution is born again. In the Bible it is the tentmaker, Saul of Tarsus, on the road to Damascus, becoming the apostle Paul. These stories are about a comeback, or a redemption (think Stephen King's *The Shawshank Redemption*).

JOY'S SMILE REBIRTH STORY

Here is an example of a dental comeback story:

For Joy, a hard-working woman in her late thirties, going to the dentist was a scary prospect. Joy was never fond of going to the dentist. In fact, you could say she was quite fearful. The morbid fear of dentists began when she wrecked her bicycle in the fifth grade and broke her upper centrals (front middle teeth) close to the gumline. She had two root canals and two crowns.

Due to lack of funds, coupled with the fact that Joy's parents were on a budget, Joy didn't go back to the dentist. Twenty-five years came and went, and Joy's dental health deteriorated. One day she was eating popcorn and felt a snap. One of her teeth, under the crown, broke at the gum line. Joy now found herself snaggletoothed. She was beyond embarrassed and hardly smiled anymore. She knew she had to go to the dentist and was not only anxious about the dental treatment, she also knew she likely had a lot of needed treatment. With her work schedule, it would be difficult managing all of the time away from the office. Joy spoke with her sister, Beth, who also shared Joy's fear of dental treatment. Beth said her dentist not only did great work, but also could do something called sedation dentistry. Beth had been in recently for multiple procedures, was sedated, and had everything done in one visit. Best of all, she practically slept through it. Joy had never been so excited to call a dental office. She made the call and booked an evaluation. Joy's smile was reborn.

Not only did Joy complete her treatment in two appointments, she also utilized a patient financing option from CareCredit and was able to spread her payments over thirty-six months. Joy tells everyone she knows, if she knew that taking care of her teeth could be that simple, she would have had them fixed a long time ago.

Here are some classic examples:

A *Christmas Carol* (story by Charles Dickens and many film versions). On Christmas Eve, crotchety miser Ebenezer Scrooge (main character) is visited by the ghost of his dead partner Jacob Marley. Scrooge is told that what they do in life will determine what happens to them in the afterlife. Marley tells Scrooge that he will be visited by three ghosts (mentor characters) and to take heed of what happens. The first spirit, the Ghost of Christmas Past, shows Scrooge that he was once a happy young man, carefree and in love, but money became his greatest desire. The Ghost of Christmas Present shows him how others, including his nephew Fred and his clerk Bob Cratchit, are spending a poor but loving holiday together, as well as Tiny Tim's crutch by a fireplace. The Ghost of Christmas Yet to Come shows Scrooge the fate that awaits him. Scrooge learns from his visits and becomes a good man who knows how to celebrate Christmas as well as how to live better the rest of the year.

The Parable of the Prodigal Son (from the Christian Greek scriptures of the Bible, Luke 15). The story was told by arguably the greatest teacher (and storyteller) who ever lived, Jesus of Nazareth. In the story, a father has two sons. The younger son asks for his inheritance before the father dies, and the father agrees. The younger son, after wasting his fortune (the word "prodigal" means "wastefully extravagant"), goes hungry during a famine, and becomes so destitute he longs to eat the same food given to hogs, which are unclean animals in Jewish culture. He then returns home with the intention of repenting and begging his father to be made one of his hired servants, expecting his relationship with his father is likely severed. Regardless, the father finds him on the road and immediately welcomes him back as his son and holds a feast to celebrate his return, which includes killing a fattened calf usually reserved for special occasions. The older son refuses to participate, stating that in all the time he has worked for the father, he never disobeyed him; yet, he did not even receive a goat to celebrate with his friends. The father reminds the older son that the son has always been with him and everything the father has belongs to the older son (his inheritance). But they should still celebrate the return of the younger son because he was lost and is now found. (That is where the story ends. We do not know if the older brother, who was righteous in his indignation, forgave his brother and joined the celebration. How do you think the story should end?)

The Natural (a movie by Barry Levinson; based on a novel by Bernard Malmaud). Here is the long plot synopsis. The movie opens with a young farm boy, Roy Hobbs (main character), who has an incredible talent for playing baseball. Encouraged by his father, Hobbs is told by him that he has an amazing gift for throwing a baseball, but he needs more than that if he is to succeed and play in the big leagues. Hobbs witnesses his father's death; he dies while working under a large tree in the front of his home. Some years later, a lightning bolt strikes the tree, splitting it into pieces. Hobbs takes a part of the tree and carves out a bat, using a tool to burn into the bat the name Wonderboy, along with a symbol of a lightning bolt for whence it came.

A few years later, Hobbs finds out he is going to get a chance to play in the big leagues. In the middle of the night, he runs to meet his longtime girlfriend, Iris Gaines (mentor), to inform her that he is going to try out for the Chicago Cubs. When he arrives in Chicago, a woman asks Hobbs to confirm what he told her on the train; that he would eventually be the best in the game. When Hobbs agrees, she raises a gun and shoots him.

Fifteen years later, Pop Fisher, the manager of the New York Knights, discovers he has a new "rookie" for his team, a thirty-four-year-old man named Roy Hobbs, whom the team's owner, the stingy Judge Banner (nemesis), has signed for a paltry $500. The Knights begin to rise in the standings due to Hobbs's amazing performance. The lightning bolt on his bat inspires teammates. Soon after, the entire team adopts the lightning bolt patch, which is worn on their right sleeves. The team's stellar hitting continues, as does the win streak for the Knights. While getting a shoeshine one afternoon, a coach tells Hobbs about the deal that the judge made with Pop to swindle the remaining shares from him. If Pop wins the pennant, the Judge would give away his shares. If Pop loses, then the judge gets all of Pop's shares and he's out for good.

After the game, Hobbs receives a note from Iris requesting to meet with him. Hobbs meets Iris at a café, where they have a cordial visit. Upon leaving, Hobbs asks Iris to come to the next game, but she says she can't for other reasons. After another great game performance, Hobbs leaves the ballpark only to find Iris waiting for him outside. The two walk to her home from the ballpark. During the walk, Hobbs elaborates to Iris about his troubled past and why he failed to return for Iris after leaving for Chicago. At her home, Hobbs notices a baseball glove on the couch. Iris informs him it belongs to her son. Hobbs is shocked to hear this and asks where the father is. Iris says that his father lives in New York (Roy is a little slow on the uptake here).

Hobbs regains his focus, as do the rest of the Knights, and the team begins a winning streak that results in the Knights being three games ahead of the Pirates in the standings for the pennant with just three games to go. The Knights hold a banquet for the team. Confederates of the judge poison the unsuspecting Hobbs with a tainted piece of food. This results in Hobbs being taken to a local hospital where he is laid up sick for three days. During his visit, the doctor informs Hobbs that his stomach lining has been gradually deteriorating. Upon pumping his stomach, the doctors remove an old bullet that had apparently been there for years. He is warned if he ever plays baseball again, it may be fatal.

Meanwhile, the Knights lose their next three games, allowing the Pirates to catch up and tie with them for first place. Judge Banner visits Hobbs and offers him $20,000 to throw the next game, which will decide who wins the pennant. The judge leaves Hobbs with the money, assuming that they have a deal.

Iris comes to visit Hobbs at the hospital. Hobbs admits to his failure of falling for the woman on the train all those years ago, and how all of that resulted in his life not turning out how he expected. Hobbs returns to the ballpark the next day, gives the Judge back his envelope of money, informing them all that it's his plan to play in the game that evening.

Hobbs hits a walk-off homer to win the game and pennant. As the team jumps on Hobbs as he crosses home plate, the camera pans to the ball that is still flying out into the night. Cut to Iris's farm. As the ball drops in the next sequence, it lands in the glove of Iris's son, who throws the ball back to his father, Roy Hobbs, as Iris lovingly looks on.

HOW TO APPLY THE REBIRTH STORY

A rebirth story is about something that was doomed making a comeback. In a rebirth story the main character is at the bottom and then rises from the depths. This is similar to an underdog story, but the main character in a rebirth story does not need to be alone in the world like the underdog character (if the main character is an orphan, you can bet it is an underdog story).

Wendy's Rebirth Story

By Debra Engelhardt Nash

Wendy had just come from another dental office when she walked into the reception room. She was a lovely woman (we later found out she was a model). But today she looked anxious. A bit teary-eyed, she confessed: "I don't have an appointment."

She explained she and her husband did not have insurance, so they called around looking for an office with low fees and found a coupon special from another practice offering an exam at an affordable price. She made an appointment to have her teeth cleaned and examined on this day—the day she was sitting in front of me.

Wendy proceeded to tell me that when she went in she was told she could not have a standard cleaning that day because she had periodontal disease. She was also told she needed to have her wisdom teeth extracted soon and she had eight cavities. Wendy said she was stunned. She asked for her treatment plan and her x-rays and told them she would get back with them.

She got in her car and started to cry. Then she called her husband.

He told her that when he was telephone shopping he spoke to a nice woman in an office and although he didn't know what would happen, he suggested to his wife that she stop in that practice on her way home. So, Wendy did. And she was sitting in front of the person who had taken her husband's call: me.

I excused myself for a moment and went back to speak to one of our hygienists. I asked if she had a few moments to see the person in the reception room. Since our office has a can-do attitude, she said, "Of course."

I introduced her to Wendy and she was escorted back to the treatment area.

In a few moments, the hygienist came out and said, "I don't find perio. Her tissue is healthier than mine." We then went to Dr. Nash to tell him what was going on and he proceeded to come into the operatory to meet Wendy.

Dr. Nash reviewed her x-rays, did an oral exam, and stated she should have her wisdom teeth out at some time, but he didn't find any cavities or perio disease. Wendy had tears of joy.

Dr. Nash asked the hygienist if she could make time to clean Wendy's teeth. When Wendy inquired about the fee, Dr Nash said, "You already paid for it."

Wendy replied, "But I paid the other office."

Dr Nash responded, "I know. You already paid for it."

More tears of appreciation.

Wendy did have her teeth cleaned that day. Dr. Nash also spoke to her about how he could improve her smile, although it was already lovely. He wanted her to know there were cosmetic improvement and treatment possibilities and discussed them with her.

The patient who had initially been shopping for the lowest fee to have her teeth cleaned decided instead she would like to have veneers, and chose to afford ten porcelain veneers for her anterior teeth. Wendy and her husband were shopping for low fees, but after learning what's possible, found cosmetic dentistry affordable.

Wendy's modeling career began to flourish. At our encouragement, she entered the Mrs. North Carolina pageant and won, and she was first runner-up in the Mrs. America pageant.

Wendy's life was changed. And when you see Wendy in one of the many catalogs or national advertisements, you will see a happy, successful woman with a beautiful smile.

Here's the moral of the story: Never assume the patient isn't interested in the best treatment you choose to offer. If they don't know what's possible, they will never choose it. Always offer the best care and help your patients choose what's right for them.

[CHAPTER 12]
ESCAPE STORIES

Many films have "escape" right in the title: *Escape from New York, The Great Escape,* and *Escape from Witch Mountain* come to mind. An escape story starts in a normal place, goes to a crazy place, and then the characters must cheat death and make it back to a normal place: home. As Glinda the Good Witch teaches Dorothy Gale in Oz, there's no place like home (could have used that advice when the house landed on the first witch, but oh well).

Here are some examples:

The Time Machine (story by H.G. Wells and adapted into several films). Alexander Hartdegen (main character) is a scientist and an inventor who is determined to prove that time travel is possible. When the girl he loves is tragically killed, Alexander is determined to go back in time and change the past. Testing his theories, the time machine is hurtled 800,000 years into the future. He discovers a terrifying new world. Instead of mankind being the hunter, they are now the hunted, with him stuck in the middle. He must escape the future and get back to his own time.

Gone with the Wind (novel by Margaret Mitchell and film produced by David O. Selznick). This epic tale of the Old South from the start of the Civil War through to the period of reconstruction focuses on the beautiful Scarlett O'Hara (main character). This story is about escaping the ravages of war. Before the start of the war, life at the O'Hara plantation, Tara, could only be described as genteel (except, of course, if you were a slave). As for the young Scarlett, she is without doubt the most beautiful girl in the area. She is looking forward to a barbecue at the nearby Wilkes plantation, as she will get to see the man she loves, Ashley Wilkes. She is more than a little dismayed when she hears that he is to marry his cousin, Melanie Hamilton, and in a fit of anger, she decides to marry Melanie's brother. The Civil War (nemesis) is soon declared and as always seems to be the case, men march off to battle thinking that it will only last a few weeks. Now living in Atlanta, Scarlett sees the ravages that war brings. She also becomes reacquainted with Rhett Butler (later the mentor character), whom she had first met at the Wilkes barbecue. Now a widow, she still pines for the married Ashley and dreams of his return. With the war lost, however, she returns to Tara and faces the hardship of keeping her family together and Tara from being sold at auction to collect the taxes. She has become hardened and bitter and will do anything, including marrying her sister's beau, to ensure "with God as my witness" she will never again be poor and hungry. After becoming a widow for the second time, she finally marries the dashing Rhett, but they soon find themselves working at cross-purposes, their relationship seemingly doomed from the outset. Rhett leaves with a classic "Oh, snap" exit line. Scarlett realizes that even if she doesn't get Rhett back, she can always return to the land—to escape back to Tara. As Scarlett says: "Tara! Home. I'll go home, and I'll think of some way to get him back! After all, tomorrow is another day!"

HOW TO APPLY THE ESCAPE STORY

The escape story is about being in a normal place, going to a crazy place, and getting back to normal. You are telling how the hero escaped a bad situation. This is similar to the rebirth story. Here is an example.

One of our other patients, Jim, found himself in a situation that's similar to yours. Jim once had a good job and good teeth. But he fell upon rocky times. Jim had the undeserved misfortune of being unemployed, and that can be hard to escape. Then an opportunity came along, but it would not be easy. After years of neglect due to a lack of funds to take care of his dental needs, Jim found himself in quite a dilemma. He had a job offer as a blackjack dealer in a new casino. But the casino hiring manager had given him a couple of demands before he could begin the job.

"First, get a haircut, and second, get those teeth fixed," said the manager at the casino.

The haircut was an easy task. The second request was a bit more daunting. Jim needed the income from the job to get his teeth fixed, and he couldn't secure the job until he had a plan to have his teeth fixed. Because he had been unemployed for a while, Jim didn't qualify for patient financing.

Here was the good news. Jim's employer said he could begin training while he was having his smile restored. The training program was twelve weeks. The dentist had advice to share with Jim. He offered a payment arrangement where Jim could prepay, making weekly payments and when he was 75 percent paid, the office would schedule him a week or two out for his extractions and immediate dentures.

Jim was so motivated and had such a clear picture of what he wanted for himself that the plan worked amazingly well. What was the end result? In twelve weeks, Jim not only had his work completed but he also came in for one of his post-op denture adjustments. It was not only the haircut and the new smile that made the difference, it was Jim's newfound sense of confidence.

That is how Jim escaped unemployment. If Jim's story resonates with you, we would love to put together a plan to help you get the smile that you are wanting.

[APPENDIX A]
CONVERSATION EXPERT KATHERINE EITEL BELT

**How To Have Courageous Conversations
That Lead To Case Acceptance**

Conversations can attract or repel patients.

We've all done it: Avoiding patient conversations we *need* to have because we're afraid.

"We may have spoken to someone in the past with the best of intentions and when those conversations did not go well, we learned to avoid them," says Katherine Eitel Belt. "The problem with avoiding, of course, is that situations rarely resolve themselves and typically get worse over time, which only strengthens our irritation, confusion, or negative feelings, and erodes openness, creativity, and weakens relationships."

Belt runs a company called LionSpeak Communications Coaching. She advises that a dentist can engage in conversations with predictably better outcomes by recognizing and shifting limiting beliefs and adding a few of these tools:

I never lose. I either win or I learn. "When you believe you cannot lose, no matter how the conversation goes, and the only reality is that you will either have a good outcome for both parties or learn something powerful about what works or what doesn't, you have more courage."

Crucial information may be missing. "Listen first, talk second. 'Sara, I want to talk to you about how we are handling our end-of-day closing process. I have some concerns about it but first, I'm wondering how you think we're doing.' It's amazing the enlightening information you learn which can shift your perspective, heighten empathy, or causes you to change your mind completely."

Agreement is a good place to start. "Where you agree is a much stronger platform from which to launch the conversation. 'Would it be fair to say, Sara, that we both want to get out of here as close to 5:00 as possible to get home to our families?' Most reasonable people will agree. The rest of the conversation will be easier because it now seems in service to the foundational place of agreement."

Judgment is a relationship killer. "Very few things are actually good or bad, or right or wrong. Most either work or don't work. Instead of speaking about things being wrong or bad, switch to 'This doesn't work for maintaining our value of excellent service.' Or 'This works better for supporting the team in accomplishing our goals.'"

Belt says the world needs more non-judgmental, thoughtful, and courageous conversations.

"Open your mind and your heart," says Belt.

A great way to shift the conversation is to ask, "May I tell you a case acceptance story about someone who was in a similar situation to where you are?"

[APPENDIX B]
ACKNOWLEDGMENTS

FROM PENNY REED. It seems like only yesterday that I sat in the consultation room in our dental office and watched as Dr. David Ijams began his treatment presentations with a carousel of slides and a story of a dental patient receiving the smile of her dreams. At the time, I had no idea of the true power of that conversation. Thank you, David, for your example and for your belief in me as your dental office manager. I will always be grateful for the doors you opened for me.

Thank you to Mark LeBlanc and Henry DeVries, my coauthors and friends, whom it was a pleasure to partner with on this book. It's my hope that many, many patients achieve their goals for their smiles and oral health, because have a better understanding of optimal dental care thanks to the storytelling expertise of their dentists..

To my sweet and supportive husband Rob: thank you for your support and belief in my work. And to our girls, Brooke and Savanah, thank you for keeping me young and reminding me that it's more than okay to be myself in all that I do.

FROM HENRY DEVRIES. I want to thank the authors I have worked with as an editor and publisher who introduced me to the world of dentistry, including Alan Stern, DDS; Robert Tripke, DMD; Tija Hunter; Kevin Henry; and Penny Reed. I also want to thank experts from the dental consulting world who were helpful sources for my forbes.com column, including Paul Homoly, DDS; Minal Sampat; Vanessa Emerson; and Katherine Eitel Belt. Gratitude to my parents for taking me to the dentist when I was growing up every six years, whether I needed it or not (seriously, thanks for the braces Mom and Dad). Last but not least, I want to express thanks to my dentist Curtis E. McRae, DDS, and my rock star registered dental hygienist, Wendy Tweed, for being trusted members of my family's healthcare team.

FROM MARK LEBLANC. I want to acknowledge Katherine Eitel Belt (of LionSpeak) and Vanessa Emerson (The Dental Speakers Institute) for introducing me to the dental community.

ABOUT THE AUTHORS

Penny Reed is the founder and president of the Dental Coaching Institute, Inc. She works with dental teams who want to raise the bar on their performance and create an office culture where the entire team looks forward to coming to work every day. As a speaker, she teaches dental audiences how to grow their practices by 25 percent or more. In fact, she wrote the book, *Growing Your Dental Business*.

Reed began her career in dental office management in 1992. She discovered a passion for helping others grow their practices and has been coaching dentists and their teams since 1994. She has been named a Leader in Dental Consulting by *Dentistry Today* from 2007 to 2020. She is a member of the National

Speakers' Association, the Academy of Dental Management Consultants, and the American Association of Dental Office Management. Reed is the creator and host of the podcast "Growing Your Dental Business" on iTunes.

Reed lives in Tennessee with her husband Rob and is the proud mom of Brooke and Savanah. She has an addiction to the Disney theme parks and is always planning her next trip or dental retreat near the magic.

You can invite her to speak or talk shop about dentistry or Disney by emailing penny@dentalcoachinginstitute.com or calling 888-877-5648.

Henry DeVries is the CEO (chief encouragement officer) of Indie Books International, a company he cofounded in 2014 with Mark LeBlanc. He works with independent consultants who want to attract more high-paying clients by marketing with a book and speech. As a speaker, he trains business leaders how to sell more services by persuading with a story. In the last ten years, he has helped ghostwrite, edit, and coauthor more than 300 dental and business advice books, including his McGraw-Hill bestseller, *How to Close a Deal Like Warren Buffett*—now in five languages, including Chinese. He has authored or coauthored twelve marketing books and writes a weekly column for Forbes.com.

As a result of working with him, professionals, consultants, and business leaders report they have more impact and influence.

On a personal note, he is a baseball nut. A former Associated Press sportswriter, he has visited forty-three major league ball parks and has three to go before he "touches 'em all." His hobby is writing comedy screenplays that he plans will one day be made into films. You can invite him to speak about persuading with a case acceptance story or go to a baseball game by emailing henry@indiebooksintl.com or calling 619-540-3031.

Mark LeBlanc, CSP runs a speaking business in Minneapolis. He conducts presentations and creates experiences for independent and practice professionals who want to create an extreme sliver of focus and put more money in their pocket as a business owner. His nationally renowned *Achievers Circle* weekend business retreat is ideal for business owners who want to develop a path and plan for true business growth. The *Achievers Circle* (open enrollment) can also be tailored for a private practice and team experience.

In fact, he has authored or coauthored four business books, including *Growing Your Business, Never Be the Same, Build Your Consulting Practice* (with Henry DeVries), and *Defining YOU* (with Henry DeVries and Kathy McAfee). He has clocked over 20,000 business coaching hours, given over 1,000 presentations, and conducted over 150 business retreats. He is a past president of the National Speakers Association and a CSP or Certified Speaking Professional.

As a result of his work, people often share they are more focused each day, generate undeniable momentum, and achieve more balance between their home and work life.

LeBlanc's keynote speech and book *Never Be the Same* were inspired by walking the 500-mile Camino de Santiago pilgrimage across northern Spain. Audiences have been captivated by the self-management and self-leadership lessons learned along the trek. He is the founder of The Mark LeBlanc (Young Entrepreneurs Succeed) Foundation. The purpose is to give $3,000 grants to entrepreneurs under thirty years of age.

Find out more about him at MarkLeBlanc. com. He can be reached by emailing Mark@ GrowingYourBusiness.com or calling 612-860-9138.

[APPENDIX D]
REFERENCES

Escalas, Jennifer Edson. "Self-Referencing and Persuasion: Narrative Transportation versus Analytical Elaboration." *Journal of Consumer Research*, March 2007, Volume 33, Issue 4.

Green, Melanie, Garst, Jennifer, Brock, Timothy, and Chung Sungeun. "Fact versus Fiction Labeling: Persuasion Parity Despite Heightened Scrutiny of Fact." *Journal of Media Psychology*. 2006. Volume 8, Issue 3.

Made in the USA
Coppell, TX
29 September 2021

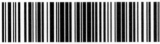